HEPATITIS DIET COOKBOOK

TABLE OF CONTENTS

CONCLUSION

INTRODUCTION

The liver, that unsung hero of our body, performs countless vital functions silently and diligently. From detoxifying the blood to metabolizing nutrients and regulating cholesterol levels, it's a multitasking marvel that often goes unnoticed until something goes amiss. One condition that can cast a spotlight on the liver's importance is hepatitis, a group of inflammatory liver diseases that can range from mild to severe and acute to chronic. If you or a loved one are grappling with hepatitis, you're already well aware of how essential it is to provide your liver with the support it needs to heal and thrive.

This is where the "Hepatitis Diet Cookbook" steps in, serving as your trusted companion on your journey to better liver health and overall well-being. Hepatitis is a complex condition, and its management requires a holistic approach that extends beyond medical treatment. Diet plays a pivotal role in this approach, and this cookbook is your gateway to harnessing the healing power of food.

The journey of crafting this cookbook began with a recognition of the challenges that individuals living with hepatitis face. These challenges include the physical toll on the body and the emotional and psychological impact of a diagnosis. Whether you're navigating Hepatitis A, B, C, or another variation, it's a journey fraught with questions, uncertainties, and the quest for a balanced and wholesome diet that supports your liver's healing process.

- UNDERSTANDING HEPATITIS

Hepatitis is a term that refers to the inflammation of the liver. It is a condition that can have various causes, with viral infections being the most common. Understanding hepatitis is crucial because it affects millions of people worldwide and can lead to serious health complications if left untreated.

Symptoms:

Symptoms of hepatitis can range from mild to severe and may include:

- Jaundice (yellowing of the skin and eyes)

- Fatigue

- Abdominal pain

- Nausea and vomiting

- Loss of appetite

- Dark urine

- Clay-colored stools

- Joint pain

- Fever

- Itchy skin

It's important to note that some people with hepatitis may remain asymptomatic for years, unknowingly carrying the virus and potentially spreading it to others.

PREVENTION AND MANAGEMENT:

Preventing hepatitis is crucial, especially for viral forms of the disease. Vaccines are available for hepatitis A and hepatitis B and are recommended for those at risk. Preventive measures also include practicing safe sex, avoiding sharing needles, and practicing good hygiene, such as handwashing.

For those living with chronic hepatitis, management is essential. Antiviral medications are available for hepatitis B and C, which can help suppress the virus and reduce the risk of complications. Lifestyle changes, including limiting alcohol consumption and maintaining a healthy diet, can also support liver health.

Hepatitis is a significant global health concern with various causes and potential complications. Understanding the types, causes, symptoms, and preventive measures is essential for individuals and communities to reduce the incidence of hepatitis and improve overall liver health. Early detection and proper management play a vital role in preventing long-term liver damage and complications.

- IMPORTANCE OF DIET IN HEPATITIS MANAGEMENT

The importance of diet in the management of hepatitis cannot be overstated. Hepatitis, a condition characterized by inflammation of the liver, can have a profound impact on one's overall health and well-being. Diet plays a crucial role in mitigating the symptoms, supporting liver function, and aiding in the recovery process. Here's why dietary choices are of paramount significance in hepatitis management:

1. Liver Support: The liver is the body's primary detoxifying organ, and it plays a pivotal role in processing and eliminating toxins from the body. In hepatitis, the liver is already under stress. A well-balanced diet that is gentle on the liver can help reduce its workload, allowing it to heal and regenerate.

2. Minimizing Inflammation: Hepatitis is characterized by liver inflammation. Certain foods, such as those high in saturated fats, processed sugars, and additives, can exacerbate inflammation. Conversely, an anti-inflammatory diet rich in fruits, vegetables, and whole grains can help reduce inflammation and provide relief from discomfort.

3. Nutrient Replenishment: Hepatitis can lead to nutrient deficiencies due to impaired absorption and utilization. A diet that is rich in vitamins, minerals, and antioxidants can help replenish these essential nutrients, supporting overall health and aiding the body's immune response.

4. Weight Management: Maintaining a healthy weight is crucial for individuals with hepatitis, as excess weight can contribute to liver fat accumulation and worsen liver health. A well-planned diet can help individuals achieve and maintain a healthy weight, reducing the strain on the liver.

5. Balanced Blood Sugar Levels: Hepatitis can affect blood sugar regulation. Consuming a diet that includes complex carbohydrates, fiber, and lean proteins can help stabilize blood sugar levels, preventing energy crashes and mood swings.

6. Protein Intake: Adequate protein intake is vital for liver repair and maintenance. However, the source of protein matters. Lean proteins like poultry, fish, tofu, and legumes are easier for the liver to process than fatty cuts of meat.

7. Hydration: Proper hydration is essential for liver function and toxin elimination. Drinking Enough

water helps flush toxins out of the body and supports digestion.

HOW TO USE THIS COOKBOOK

1. Understanding Your Dietary Needs: Before diving into the recipes, take a moment to read the introductory chapters. Understanding the basics of hepatitis and dietary guidelines will empower you to make informed food choices tailored to your health needs.

2. Recipe Organization: This cookbook is thoughtfully organized into chapters, each focusing on a specific meal category, from wholesome breakfasts to satisfying main courses and delightful desserts. You can easily locate recipes based on your dietary preferences or the time of day.

3. Recipe Selection: Explore a variety of mouthwatering recipes, each designed to align with hepatitis management principles. Whether you're craving a comforting soup, a refreshing salad, or a hearty main dish, there's something for every palate.

4. Nutritional Information: Every recipe includes detailed nutritional information, such as calories, protein, and fiber content, enabling you to make

informed decisions about your diet and portion control.

5. Meal Planning: In Chapter 9, you'll find meal plans and sample menus to help you structure your eating habits. These plans offer flexibility while ensuring a balanced and hepatitis-friendly diet.

6. Cooking Tips and Techniques: Refer to Chapter 10 for valuable cooking tips and techniques, including safe food handling and kitchen tools to make your culinary journey a seamless and enjoyable experience.

7. Beyond the Plate: Remember that managing hepatitis is not solely about diet; it encompasses overall wellness. The concluding section delves into holistic approaches to living well with hepatitis, offering insights beyond the kitchen.

CHAPTER 1

BASICS OF HEPATITIS AND DIETARY GUIDELINES

- Types of Hepatitis

There are several types of hepatitis, but the most common ones are hepatitis A, B, and C:

1. Hepatitis A (HAV): Typically transmitted through contaminated food or water, hepatitis A is an acute infection that doesn't typically lead to chronic liver disease.

2. Hepatitis B (HBV): This virus can spread through contact with infected blood, bodily fluids, or from an infected mother to her newborn. Chronic hepatitis B can lead to severe liver damage.

3. Hepatitis C (HCV): Hepatitis C is primarily transmitted through contact with infected blood. It often becomes chronic and can lead to cirrhosis or liver cancer if left untreated.

Causes of Hepatitis:

Hepatitis can result from various causes, including viral infections, alcohol abuse, certain medications, and autoimmune diseases. Viral hepatitis is the most common cause and can lead to acute or chronic hepatitis, depending on the virus and individual factors.

- Hepatitis Diet: What to Include and Avoid

Managing hepatitis through a well-balanced diet is crucial for supporting liver health and minimizing the strain on this vital organ. Understanding what to include and avoid in a hepatitis diet is key to managing the condition effectively.

What to Include:

1. Lean Protein: Incorporate lean sources of protein like chicken, turkey, fish, tofu, and legumes. Protein is essential for liver repair and regeneration.

2. Fruits and Vegetables: Fresh fruits and vegetables are rich in antioxidants and fiber, which aid digestion and help the liver detoxify. Opt for a variety of colorful options.

3. Whole Grains: Whole grains like brown rice, quinoa, and whole wheat provide essential nutrients and fiber while preventing blood sugar spikes.

4. Healthy Fats: Include sources of healthy fats such as avocados, nuts, seeds, and olive oil. Omega-3 fatty acids, found in fatty fish like salmon, can reduce inflammation.

5. Dairy or Dairy Alternatives: Choose low-fat or dairy-free options for calcium and vitamin D. Yogurt with probiotics supports gut health.

What to Avoid:

1. Alcohol: Alcohol can worsen liver damage and should be completely avoided if you have hepatitis.

2. Highly Processed Foods: Foods high in refined sugars, saturated fats, and additives can strain the liver and contribute to inflammation.

3. Excessive Sodium: High sodium intake can lead to fluid retention and worsen liver-related complications. Limit salt intake.

4. Raw Seafood and Shellfish: These can carry harmful bacteria and viruses that may pose a greater risk to individuals with hepatitis.

5. Supplements and Herbal Remedies: Consult a healthcare professional before taking any

supplements or herbal remedies, as some can interact with medications or worsen liver function.

Also, a hepatitis diet should be tailored to your specific condition and treatment plan.

PORTION CONTROL AND MEAL PLANNING FOR HEPATITIS MANAGEMENT

Proper portion control and meal planning play a crucial role in managing hepatitis, as they help reduce the strain on the liver, maintain stable blood sugar levels, and support overall well-being. These dietary strategies can improve digestion, alleviate symptoms, and promote liver health for individuals living with hepatitis.

1. Portion Control:

   - Smaller, Frequent Meals: Opt for smaller, more frequent meals throughout the day to prevent overloading the liver and aid in digestion.

   - Monitor Protein Intake: Limit protein portions to avoid excess ammonia production, which the liver must process. Choose lean protein sources like poultry, fish, and tofu.

  - Mindful Eating: Pay attention to hunger and fullness cues, slowing down during meals to savor flavors and prevent overeating.

  - Reduce Sodium: Limit sodium intake to help manage fluid retention and swelling, common symptoms in hepatitis.

2. Meal Planning:

  - Balanced Diet: Plan meals that include a balance of carbohydrates, lean proteins, healthy fats, and a variety of fruits and vegetables.

  - Fiber-Rich Foods: Incorporate high-fiber foods like whole grains, legumes, and fresh produce to support digestion and prevent constipation.

  - Limit Sugar: Minimize added sugars, as excessive sugar consumption can strain the liver. Opt for natural sweeteners like honey or fresh fruits.

  - Hydration: Stay well-hydrated with water and herbal teas to aid digestion and flush out toxins.

Sample Meal Plan:

- Breakfast: Scrambled eggs with spinach and whole-grain toast.

- Snack: Greek yogurt with berries.

- Lunch: Grilled chicken salad with mixed greens, cucumbers, and a vinaigrette dressing.

- Snack: Sliced apple with almond butter.

- Dinner: Baked salmon with quinoa and steamed broccoli.

Carrying out portion control and thoughtful meal planning, individuals with hepatitis can enjoy a well-balanced diet that supports liver health, alleviates symptoms, and enhances overall quality of life. Consulting with a healthcare provider or registered dietitian can provide personalized guidance to ensure dietary choices align with specific hepatitis management needs.

CHAPTER 2

BREAKFAST DELIGHTS

Breakfast, often hailed as the most important meal of the day, takes on an even greater significance when managing hepatitis. A nutritious morning meal can set the tone for the rest of the day, providing essential nutrients, supporting liver health, and aiding digestion. In this collection of "Breakfast Delights for Hepatitis," we embark on a culinary journey that combines flavor, healing properties, and easy preparation to help individuals living with hepatitis start their day right.

Navigating hepatitis requires a holistic approach to well-being, and the choices we make at the breakfast table can significantly impact our health. This cookbook is designed to provide a range of delicious and wholesome breakfast options that cater to the unique dietary needs of those managing hepatitis. Whether you're seeking protein-packed dishes, fiber-rich options, or gentle, liver-friendly recipes, this collection has you covered.

from hearty oatmeal bowls to energizing smoothies and savory egg creations. Each recipe is thoughtfully crafted to support liver function, reduce inflammation, and promote overall wellness. Moreover, we'll delve into the importance of mindful eating, portion control, and making informed ingredient choices to enhance your breakfast routine and your liver health.

- CREAMY OATMEAL WITH FRESH BERRIES

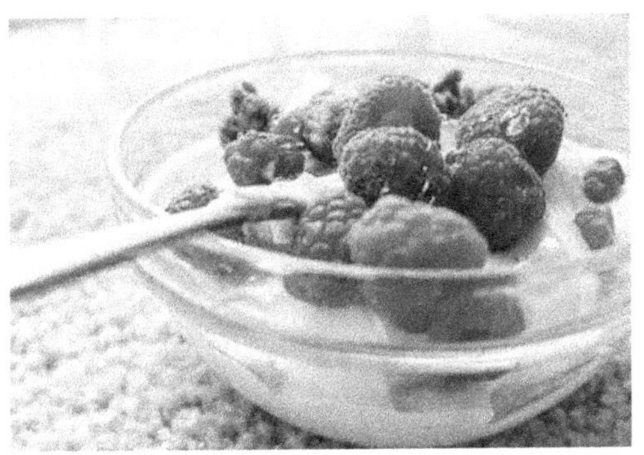

Benefits:

Creamy oatmeal with fresh berries is not only a comforting and delicious breakfast but also a powerhouse of nutrition with numerous benefits for your overall health, especially for individuals managing hepatitis.

1. Liver Support: Oats are rich in soluble fiber, which helps regulate cholesterol levels and supports liver function. A healthy liver is essential for those with hepatitis.

2. Sustained Energy: Oatmeal provides a slow release of energy, helping to stabilize blood sugar levels throughout the morning, preventing energy crashes.

3. Antioxidant Boost: Fresh berries, such as strawberries, blueberries, or raspberries, are loaded with antioxidants that combat oxidative stress and inflammation, supporting liver health.

4. Digestive Aid: Oats contain soluble fiber, which aids digestion and prevents constipation, a common concern for individuals with hepatitis.

5. Nutrient-Rich: Berries are packed with essential vitamins and minerals, including vitamin C and folate, which are crucial for immune function and overall well-being.

Preparation:

Creating creamy oatmeal with fresh berries is quick and easy:

Ingredients:

- 1/2 cup rolled oats

- 1 cup milk (or a dairy-free alternative)

- A pinch of salt

- Fresh berries (strawberries, blueberries, or raspberries)

- Honey or maple syrup (optional for sweetness)

- Chopped nuts or seeds (optional for added texture and nutrients)

Instructions:

1. Combine rolled oats, milk, and a pinch of salt in a saucepan.

2. Cook over medium heat, stirring occasionally, until the oats reach your desired consistency (usually 5-7 minutes).

3. Once cooked, transfer to a bowl and top with fresh berries.

4. Drizzle with honey or maple syrup for sweetness if desired.

5. Sprinkle with chopped nuts or seeds for added texture and nutrition.

Creamy oatmeal with fresh berries is a delightful, liver-friendly breakfast that not only tastes wonderful but also provides essential nutrients to help manage hepatitis and support overall health. Enjoying this wholesome meal regularly can be a flavorful and nutritious addition to your dietary routine.

- SCRAMBLED EGGS WITH SPINACH AND TOMATOES

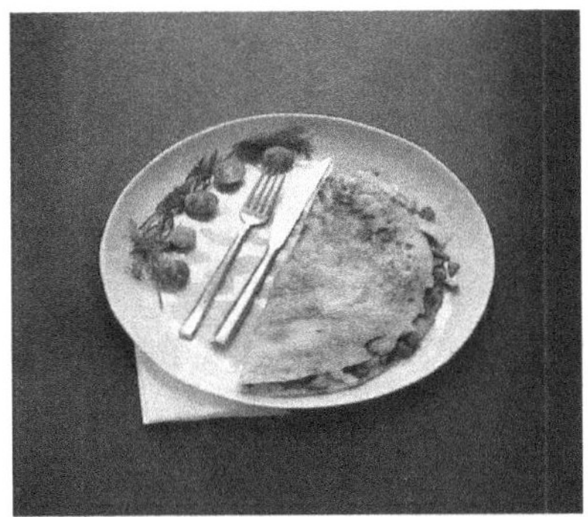

Scrambled eggs with spinach and tomatoes is not only a delicious and satisfying meal but also a nutritional powerhouse. This dish combines the protein-rich goodness of eggs with the vitamins and antioxidants found in spinach and tomatoes, making it a fantastic choice for a hearty and wholesome breakfast or brunch option.

Benefits:

1. Protein-Packed: Eggs are an excellent source of high-quality protein, which is essential for muscle maintenance, repair, and overall health.

2. Vitamins and Minerals: Spinach is rich in vitamins A, C, and K, as well as folate and iron. Tomatoes provide a dose of vitamin C and the antioxidant lycopene.

3. Low in Calories: This dish is relatively low in calories, making it a satisfying yet weight-friendly choice.

4. Fiber Content: Spinach adds dietary fiber, aiding in digestion and promoting a feeling of fullness.

Preparation:

1. Ingredients: You'll need eggs, fresh spinach leaves, ripe tomatoes, olive oil, salt, pepper, and any optional seasonings (e.g., garlic powder or paprika).

2. Sautee Spinach and Tomatoes: Heat a pan with a touch of olive oil and sauté the spinach and diced tomatoes until they soften and release their flavors.

3. Scramble Eggs: In a separate bowl, whisk the eggs with a pinch of salt and pepper. Pour the eggs into the pan with the spinach and tomatoes.

4. Cook Gently: Cook over low to medium heat, gently stirring the mixture until the eggs are just set.

5. Serve: Plate your scrambled eggs with spinach and tomatoes, adding extra seasoning or herbs if desired.

This delightful dish not only tantalizes the taste buds but also provides a nutrient-rich start to your day, offering a burst of essential vitamins, minerals, and protein. Whether enjoyed on its own or as a filling for a breakfast burrito, it's a versatile and health-conscious choice for a wholesome meal.

- CHIA PUDDING WITH MANGO

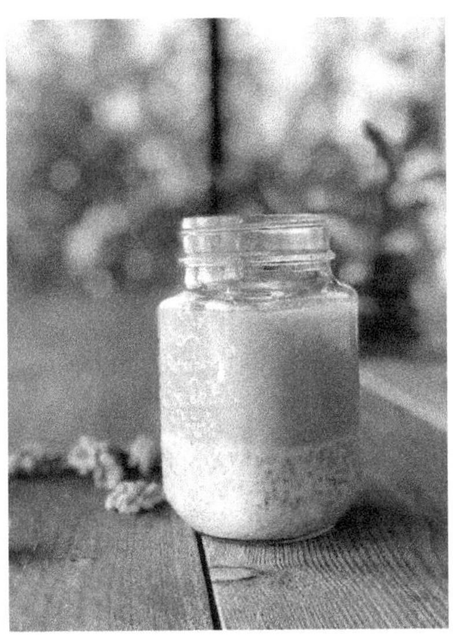

Chia pudding with mango is a delicious and nutritious treat that not only satisfies your taste buds but also provides a myriad of health benefits. This delightful dish combines the richness of chia seeds with the tropical sweetness of mango, creating a harmonious blend of flavors and textures.

Benefits:

1. Rich in Omega-3 Fatty Acids: Chia seeds are a superb source of omega-3 fatty acids, which support heart health, reduce inflammation, and promote cognitive function.

2. High in Fiber: Chia seeds are packed with dietary fiber, aiding digestion, promoting satiety, and regulating blood sugar levels.

3. Loaded with Antioxidants: Mangoes are brimming with antioxidants like vitamins A and C, which help combat free radicals and boost the immune system.

4. Nutrient-Dense: Chia seeds and mangoes offer essential vitamins, minerals, and plant compounds that contribute to overall well-being.

Preparation:

Creating chia pudding with mango is a breeze:

1. Ingredients: You'll need chia seeds, milk (dairy or plant-based), a ripe mango, a touch of honey or maple syrup for sweetness, and a pinch of vanilla extract.

2. Mix: Combine 1/4 cup of chia seeds with 1 cup of milk, a teaspoon of sweetener, and a dash of vanilla extract. Stir well and refrigerate for a few hours or overnight.

3. Blend the Mango: Puree the ripe mango in a blender until smooth.

4. Layer: In a glass or bowl, alternate layers of chia pudding and mango puree.

5. Top: Garnish with fresh mango chunks, a sprinkle of chia seeds, and a drizzle of honey or maple syrup.

Chia pudding with mango not only delights your taste buds but also nourishes your body with essential nutrients. It's a versatile dish that can be enjoyed as a wholesome breakfast, a satisfying dessert, or a nutritious snack, making it a versatile addition to a healthy diet.

- HEALING SMOOTHIE RECIPES

Smoothies are not just delicious and refreshing; they can also be powerful tools for healing and promoting overall well-being. Packed with essential nutrients, vitamins, and antioxidants, healing smoothies offer numerous health benefits while tantalizing your taste buds.

1. Immune-Boosting Berry Blast:

   - Benefits: Rich in vitamin C, antioxidants, and fiber, this smoothie supports a strong immune system, fights inflammation, and aids digestion.

   - Preparation: Blend together a cup of mixed berries (strawberries, blueberries, raspberries), a banana, Greek yogurt, and a splash of almond milk. Add honey for sweetness if desired.

2. Green Detox Elixir:

   - Benefits: Packed with leafy greens, this smoothie helps detoxify the body, boosts energy, and provides a myriad of vitamins and minerals.

   - Preparation: Blend spinach, kale, cucumber, a green apple, lemon juice, and a small piece of ginger with water or coconut water for a refreshing and cleansing drink.

3. Anti-Inflammatory Turmeric Dream:

   - Benefits: Turmeric is known for its anti-inflammatory properties. This smoothie can help reduce inflammation and alleviate joint pain.

- Preparation: Combine a frozen banana, a teaspoon of turmeric powder, a pinch of black pepper (enhances turmeric absorption), Greek yogurt, and almond milk. Add a drizzle of honey for sweetness.

4. Gut-Healing Probiotic Delight:

- Benefits: Probiotic-rich yogurt aids digestion and supports a healthy gut microbiome.

- Preparation: Blend kefir or yogurt with a banana, a handful of frozen mango chunks, and a spoonful of honey. Optionally, add a scoop of probiotic powder for an extra boost.

5. Energizing Nut Butter Bliss:

- Benefits: Loaded with protein, healthy fats, and fiber, this smoothie provides sustained energy and helps maintain blood sugar levels.

- Preparation: Mix almond or peanut butter, a banana, oats, a tablespoon of flaxseed or chia seeds, and almond milk. You can also add a touch of cinnamon for flavor.

CHAPTER 3

LIGHT AND NOURISHING SOUPS

Light and nourishing soups serve as a comforting and therapeutic addition to their dietary regimen. These soothing concoctions offer a wealth of benefits that can aid digestion, alleviate symptoms, and promote liver health while providing much-needed nourishment.

Benefits:

1. Gentle on the Liver: Hepatitis can make the liver sensitive, and rich, heavy meals may exacerbate discomfort. Light soups are easy to digest, reducing the strain on the liver.

2. Hydration: Soups contain water, which helps maintain proper hydration, a vital factor in liver function. Adequate hydration supports the liver's ability to detoxify the body.

3. Nutrient Density: Well-balanced soups can be packed with essential vitamins, minerals, and antioxidants from vegetables, lean proteins, and herbs, providing nourishment without overwhelming the digestive system.

4. Digestive Comfort: The warmth and fluidity of soups can ease digestive discomfort, reduce bloating, and prevent constipation, common concerns for those with hepatitis.

Preparation:

- Choose a Broth Base: Begin with a clear, low-sodium broth such as chicken, vegetable, or bone broth as the foundation.

- Add Lean Proteins: Incorporate lean proteins like chicken, turkey, or tofu for a protein boost that's gentle on the liver.

- Veggies Galore: Load up on nutrient-rich vegetables like carrots, zucchini, and spinach, which offer vitamins and antioxidants.

- Herbs and Spices: Flavor your soup with herbs like parsley, cilantro, and ginger, which can support liver health and digestion.

- Avoid Excess Fat: Minimize added fats like butter or heavy cream, as they can be harder to digest.

A simple yet nourishing recipe might include a chicken and vegetable broth with ginger and a medley of colorful vegetables. This combination provides essential nutrients, supports liver function, and offers comfort and relief to those managing hepatitis. Always consult with a healthcare provider or a registered dietitian for personalized dietary recommendations tailored to your specific hepatitis management needs.

- VEGETABLE BROTH WITH GINGER

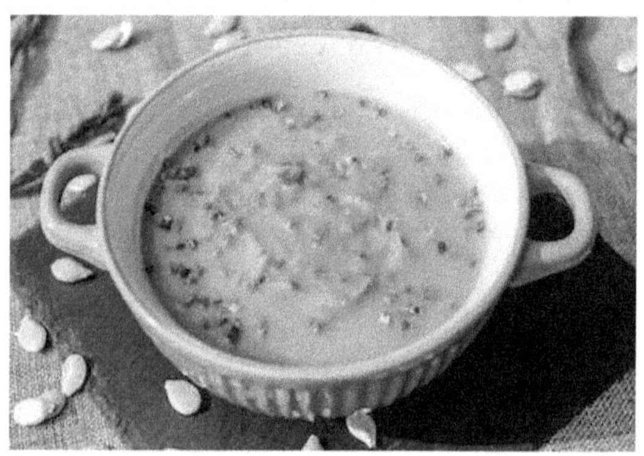

Vegetable broth with ginger is a culinary gem that combines the healing power of vegetables with the aromatic warmth of ginger. This wholesome elixir offers a multitude of benefits, making it a staple in many diets, especially for those seeking to enhance their well-being.

Benefits:

1. Digestive Support: Ginger, a well-known digestive aid, lends its soothing properties to this

broth. It can alleviate nausea, ease indigestion, and promote overall digestive health.

2. Anti-Inflammatory: The combination of vegetables and ginger provides a rich source of anti-inflammatory compounds. Regular consumption may help reduce inflammation in the body, contributing to improved health.

3. Hydration: Vegetable broth is an excellent way to stay hydrated while infusing your body with essential nutrients. Staying well-hydrated is vital for overall health.

4. Immune Boost: The vitamins, minerals, and antioxidants in vegetable broth, combined with ginger's immune-boosting properties, can help fortify your immune system, aiding in illness prevention.

Preparation:

Creating vegetable broth with ginger is a straightforward process:

- Ingredients: Gather an assortment of vegetables like carrots, celery, onions, and garlic. Add fresh ginger slices and season with herbs such as thyme and bay leaves.

- Simmer: Combine the ingredients in a large pot, cover with water, and bring to a boil. Reduce the heat and simmer for about an hour, allowing the flavors to meld.

- Strain and Enjoy: Strain the broth, discarding the solids. Your aromatic and flavorful vegetable broth with ginger is now ready to be sipped as a soothing drink, used as a base for soups, or as a cooking liquid to infuse dishes with its wonderful taste and health benefits.

Whether sipped as a comforting beverage or used as a versatile cooking ingredient, vegetable broth with ginger is a nourishing addition to any diet, offering a host of health advantages while tantalizing the taste buds with its delightful, warming flavors.

- LENTIL AND SPINACH SOUP

Lentil and Spinach Soup is a hearty, wholesome dish that not only tantalizes the taste buds but also offers a multitude of health benefits. Packed with plant-based protein, fiber, vitamins, and minerals, this soup is a nourishing choice for those seeking to support their well-being.

Benefits:

- Rich in Plant Protein: Lentils are a fantastic source of plant-based protein, which is essential for muscle maintenance and overall health. For individuals managing hepatitis, a protein-rich diet can be beneficial without overburdening the liver.

- Fiber for Digestion: Lentils and spinach are high in dietary fiber, aiding digestion and preventing constipation, a common concern for those with liver conditions.

- Abundant Nutrients: This soup is brimming with essential nutrients, including iron, folate, vitamin K, and antioxidants. These nutrients support various bodily functions, including blood health and immune system function.

- Low in Saturated Fat: Keeping saturated fat intake low is crucial for liver health. Lentils and spinach are naturally low in saturated fat, making them ideal ingredients for a hepatitis-friendly meal.

Preparation:

1. Ingredients:

   - 1 cup dried green or brown lentils (rinsed and drained)

   - 1 onion (chopped)

   - 2 cloves garlic (minced)

   - 1 carrot (chopped)

   - 1 celery stalk (chopped)

   - 4 cups vegetable broth (low-sodium)

   - 2 cups fresh spinach leaves (chopped)

   - 1 teaspoon cumin

   - Salt and pepper to taste

2. Instructions:

   a. In a large pot, sauté the chopped onion, garlic, carrot, and celery until they soften.

   b. Add the lentils, vegetable broth, and cumin. Bring to a boil, then reduce heat and simmer for 20-25 minutes or until lentils are tender.

   c. Stir in the fresh spinach and cook for an additional 2-3 minutes until wilted.

d. Season with salt and pepper to taste.

e. Serve hot and garnish with a sprinkle of fresh herbs or a squeeze of lemon if desired.

Lentil and Spinach Soup is a flavorful, nutrient-dense option that can be easily incorporated into a hepatitis-friendly diet. Its wholesome ingredients and ease of preparation make it a go-to choice for those seeking both comfort and nutrition in a single bowl.

- CREAMY BUTTERNUT SQUASH SOUP

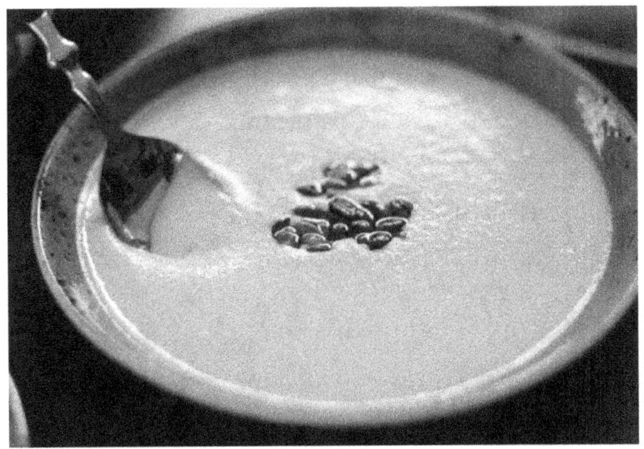

Creamy butternut squash soup is a delightful fusion of rich flavors and nourishing benefits, making it a wholesome addition to your diet, especially for those managing hepatitis. This velvety soup offers a host of advantages for liver health and overall well-being.

Benefits:

- Liver Support: Butternut squash is a superb source of antioxidants, including vitamin C and beta-carotene, which assist the liver in detoxifying the body and reducing oxidative stress.

- Digestive Comfort: The gentle, creamy texture of the soup is easy on the digestive system, making it ideal for those with hepatitis who may experience digestive challenges.

- Nutrient Density: This soup is packed with essential nutrients, such as fiber, potassium, and vitamin A, contributing to overall health and promoting regular bowel movements.

- Low in Fat: With minimal added fats, it aids in reducing excess strain on the liver, making it an excellent choice for individuals with liver conditions.

Preparation:

- Ingredients:

   - 1 medium butternut squash, peeled, seeded, and cubed

   - 1 onion, chopped

   - 2 carrots, chopped

   - 2 cloves garlic, minced

   - 4 cups vegetable broth

   - 1 teaspoon ground cinnamon

   - Salt and pepper to taste

   - Olive oil for roasting

- Instructions:

   1. Preheat your oven to 400°F (200°C).

   2. Toss the butternut squash cubes, chopped onion, and carrots with a drizzle of olive oil, salt, and pepper. Roast in the oven for about 30-35 minutes or until they're tender and slightly caramelized.

   3. In a large pot, sauté minced garlic until fragrant, then add the roasted vegetables.

4. Pour in the vegetable broth and add ground cinnamon. Bring to a simmer and cook for another 10 minutes.

5. Use an immersion blender or a countertop blender to purée the soup until smooth.

6. Season with additional salt and pepper to taste.

7. Serve hot, garnished with a sprinkle of fresh herbs or a dollop of Greek yogurt if desired.

Creamy butternut squash soup not only soothes the palate but also nurtures the body, offering a tasty way to support liver health while providing comfort and nourishment for those with hepatitis.

- HEALING CHICKEN CONGEE

Chicken congee is a time-honored and nourishing dish that has earned its place as a staple in many Asian cultures. Beyond its delightful taste, this warm and soothing porridge offers a myriad of benefits, especially for individuals seeking comfort and healing during illness or recovery.

Benefits:

- Gentle on the Stomach: Congee's soft, rice-based texture makes it easy to digest, making it ideal for those with digestive discomfort, including hepatitis patients.

- Protein-Rich: The addition of chicken provides a lean source of protein essential for tissue repair and overall health.

- Hydration: Congee is a hydrating dish, helping maintain fluid balance, which is essential for liver health.

- Nutrient Density: It's a versatile canvas for incorporating nutrient-dense ingredients such as ginger, garlic, and vegetables, each contributing to immune support and overall well-being.

Preparation:

1. Ingredients: You'll need rice (jasmine or glutinous rice for creamier congee), chicken (boneless thighs or breast), water or broth, ginger, garlic, and salt.

2. Rinse and Soak: Rinse the rice thoroughly, then soak it for about 30 minutes. This step enhances the porridge's creamy consistency.

3. Boil: In a large pot, bring the rice, chicken, and water or broth to a boil. Skim off any foam that forms on the surface.

4. Simmer: Reduce the heat to a gentle simmer. Add ginger and minced garlic for flavor and their potential health benefits.

5. Cook Slowly: Continue simmering, stirring occasionally, until the rice breaks down and the mixture thickens. This can take about 1-2 hours, depending on your desired consistency.

6. Season: Season with salt to taste.

7. Serve: Ladle the congee into bowls, and you can garnish it with green onions, cilantro, sesame oil, soy sauce, or a sprinkle of white pepper for added flavor.

CHAPTER 4

WHOLESOME SALADS

In a world increasingly conscious of health and well-being, wholesome salads have emerged as a beacon of nutrition, flavor, and vitality. These vibrant dishes are far more than just a side or appetizer; they represent a delightful journey into the world of fresh, nutrient-rich ingredients that nourish the body and tantalize the taste buds.

Wholesome salads are a celebration of nature's bounty, where colorful vegetables, crisp greens, lean proteins, and an array of delectable toppings come together in harmony. From crisp, refreshing lettuce varieties to hearty grains and legumes, these salads offer an endless canvas for creativity and culinary exploration.

But these salads are more than just a visual feast — they are a testament to the art of balancing taste and nutrition. Whether you're seeking to shed a few pounds, boost your energy, or simply embrace a healthier lifestyle, wholesome salads are your steadfast companions on the journey to better health.

In this exploration of wholesome salads, we'll delve into a world of flavors, textures, and ingredients that will elevate your dining experience. From classic favorites to innovative creations, these salads are not only satisfying but also a source of inspiration for those seeking a vibrant and health-conscious culinary adventure. So, join us on this delightful journey as we uncover the secrets of crafting and savoring the wonders of wholesome salads.

- QUINOA AND CHICKPEA SALAD

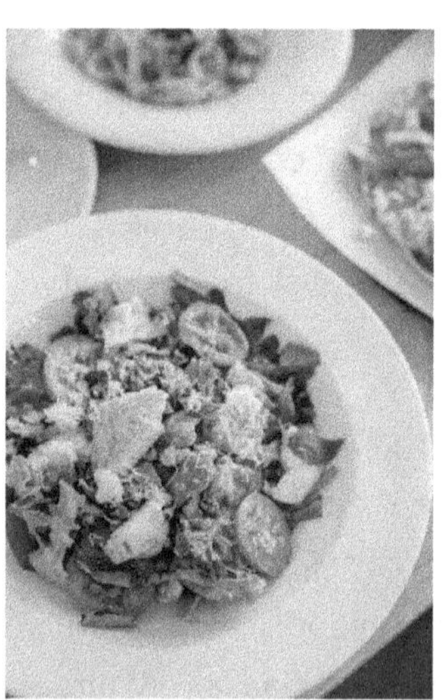

Quinoa and Chickpea Salad is a culinary gem that embodies the essence of health and taste in a single dish. This salad marries the nutty and slightly crunchy quinoa with the creamy texture and earthy flavor of chickpeas, creating a harmonious blend of flavors and textures that will delight your palate. Beyond its delectable taste, this salad boasts a multitude of health benefits, making it a staple in the repertoire of anyone seeking a nutritious and satisfying meal.

Benefits:

- Protein Powerhouse: Quinoa is a complete protein, providing all nine essential amino acids, while chickpeas are rich in plant-based protein, making this salad an excellent option for vegetarians and vegans.

- Fiber-Rich: Both quinoa and chickpeas are high in dietary fiber, aiding digestion, promoting fullness, and supporting heart health.

- Packed with Nutrients: This salad is brimming with essential vitamins and minerals, including magnesium, folate, and iron, which contribute to overall well-being.

- Gluten-Free: Quinoa is naturally gluten-free, making it suitable for those with gluten sensitivities or celiac disease.

Preparation:

- Ingredients: To prepare this salad, you'll need cooked quinoa, canned chickpeas (drained and rinsed), fresh vegetables like cucumbers and tomatoes, herbs like parsley and mint, olive oil, lemon juice, and your choice of seasonings.

- Assembly: Simply combine the cooked quinoa and chickpeas with the chopped vegetables and herbs. Drizzle with olive oil, squeeze fresh lemon juice, and season to taste with salt and pepper. Toss everything together until well-mixed.

- Versatility: You can customize your Quinoa and Chickpea Salad with additional ingredients like diced red onions, crumbled feta cheese, or a sprinkle of toasted pine nuts for added flavor and texture.

Quinoa and Chickpea Salad is not only a culinary delight but also a wholesome and satisfying dish that nourishes the body and delights the taste buds. Whether enjoyed as a main course or a side dish, this salad is a testament to the delightful synergy of health and flavor in every bite.

- BEET AND ARUGULA SALAD WITH CITRUS
DRESSING

Elevate your culinary experience and nourish your body with the delightful fusion of colors, textures, and flavors found in a Beet and Arugula Salad with Citrus Dressing. This vibrant dish not only captivates the senses but also offers a plethora of health benefits.

Benefits:

1. Rich in Nutrients: Beets are a nutritional powerhouse, packed with vitamins, minerals, and antioxidants. They support liver health, boost immunity, and promote healthy digestion.

2. Leafy Green Goodness: Arugula, the salad's base, is a leafy green known for its peppery taste and high levels of vitamins A, K, and C. It contributes to bone health, skin vitality, and overall well-being.

3. Citrus Zest: The citrus dressing adds a zingy twist to the dish. Citrus fruits, like oranges and lemons, are rich in vitamin C, which bolsters the immune

system and aids in collagen production for healthy skin.

Preparation:

Creating this salad is a breeze:

- Start by roasting or steaming the beets until tender. Allow them to cool, then peel and slice them into thin rounds or wedges.

- Combine fresh arugula with the beet slices in a salad bowl.

- For the citrus dressing, whisk together fresh orange or lemon juice, olive oil, a touch of honey or maple syrup, and a pinch of salt and pepper.

- Drizzle the dressing over the salad just before serving, and garnish with chopped fresh herbs, such as mint or basil, for an extra burst of flavor.

- AVOCADO AND TOMATO SALAD

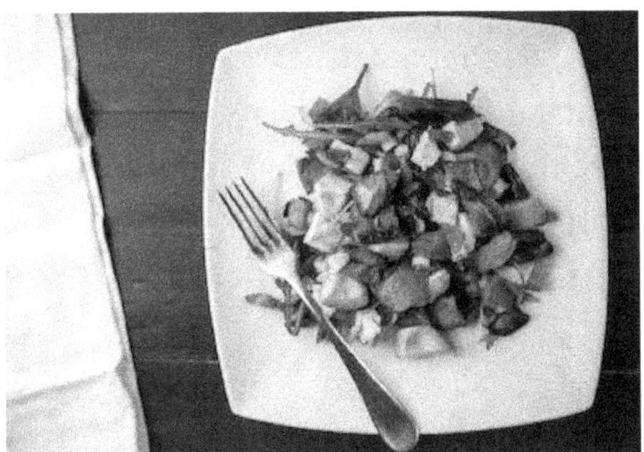

Few culinary creations exemplify the marriage of simplicity and deliciousness quite like the Avocado and Tomato Salad. This vibrant and refreshing dish has become a beloved favorite for health-conscious food enthusiasts, and it's no wonder why. The combination of creamy, nutrient-rich avocados and juicy, flavorful tomatoes creates a symphony of taste and texture that's both satisfying and beneficial for your well-being.

Benefits:

This salad isn't just a feast for your taste buds; it's a boon for your health. Avocados are renowned for their heart-healthy monounsaturated fats, which can help lower bad cholesterol levels. They also offer a generous dose of dietary fiber, potassium, and a wealth of vitamins and antioxidants. Tomatoes, on the other hand, provide lycopene, a potent antioxidant that has been linked to numerous health benefits, including reduced risk of chronic diseases.

Preparation:

Creating this salad is as straightforward as it is rewarding. Begin by slicing ripe avocados and juicy tomatoes into bite-sized pieces. Toss them together in a bowl and add a drizzle of extra-virgin olive oil, a splash of balsamic vinegar, and a sprinkle of salt and pepper to taste. Enhance the flavors with fresh herbs like basil or cilantro, and for an extra dimension of taste, consider adding ingredients like red onion, mozzarella cheese, or toasted pine nuts.

This Avocado and Tomato Salad is a versatile masterpiece that can be served as a refreshing side dish, a light meal on its own, or a nutritious accompaniment to a variety of main courses. Whether you're looking for a quick, healthy snack or a vibrant addition to your dinner table, this salad is a culinary gem that delights your palate while nourishing your body.

- PROTEIN-PACKED TUNA SALAD

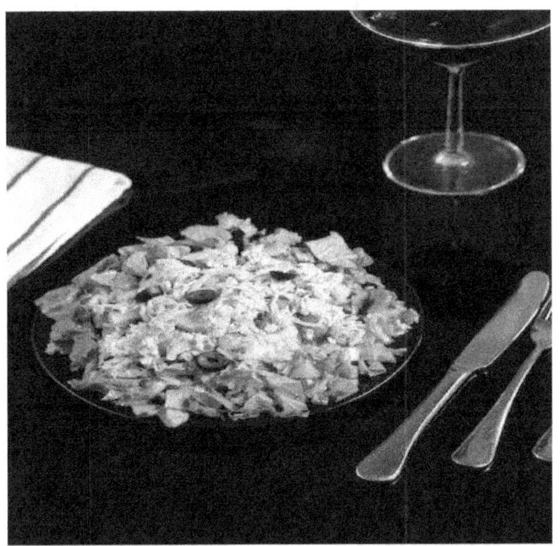

In the realm of wholesome and satisfying meals, few dishes strike the balance of taste, nutrition, and convenience as well as the Protein-Packed Tuna Salad. Renowned for its high protein content, this culinary delight has garnered a loyal following not only for its delicious taste but also for the myriad of health benefits it offers.

Benefits:

Protein Powerhouse: Tuna, the star of this salad, is a lean and protein-rich seafood that supports muscle growth and repair, making it a favorite among fitness enthusiasts.

Omega-3 Fatty Acids: Tuna is also a prime source of heart-healthy omega-3 fatty acids, which have been linked to reduced inflammation, improved cardiovascular health, and enhanced cognitive function.

Nutrient Diversity: This salad often incorporates an array of colorful vegetables, providing essential vitamins, minerals, and antioxidants that promote overall well-being and immune system support.

Weight Management: Protein helps control appetite and keeps you feeling full, making this salad a valuable addition to weight management and healthy eating plans.

Preparation:

Creating a Protein-Packed Tuna Salad is a breeze. Simply combine canned tuna (preferably packed in water for a lower calorie and fat option) with a variety of chopped vegetables such as celery, carrots, red onion, and bell peppers. Add your favorite greens like spinach or mixed lettuce for an extra nutritional boost. Flavor it with a drizzle of olive oil, a splash of lemon juice, and a pinch of salt and pepper. Customize further with ingredients like olives, capers, or avocado for added flavor and texture.

CHAPTER 5

BALANCED MAIN COURSES

In the journey towards managing hepatitis, the importance of maintaining a balanced and nutrient-rich diet cannot be overstated. As the central hub of metabolic processes in the body, the liver plays a vital role in processing nutrients, detoxifying harmful substances, and supporting overall well-being. Therefore, selecting balanced main courses is a key component of hepatic health, ensuring that the liver receives the necessary nutrients without overburdening it.

This section of our hepatitis dietary guide is dedicated to exploring a delightful array of main course options specially crafted for individuals managing hepatitis. Each dish is thoughtfully designed to strike a harmonious balance between flavor and nutrition, providing a pleasurable dining experience while promoting liver health.

From succulent baked salmon to tender grilled chicken and plant-based options like tofu stir-fry, these recipes are tailored to offer optimal nourishment for your liver. Discover how the right combination of lean proteins, whole grains, and vibrant vegetables can not only satisfy your palate but also support your journey towards hepatitis management.

As we embark on this culinary adventure, let us delve into a world of delectable and nourishing main courses, celebrating the power of balanced eating as a cornerstone of hepatic wellness.

- BAKED SALMON WITH DILL SAUCE

Baked salmon with dill sauce is a culinary masterpiece that not only tantalizes the taste buds but also offers a myriad of health benefits. This dish is a celebration of the sea's bounty, combining the rich, tender flesh of salmon with the bright, aromatic notes of dill sauce. Its preparation is a harmonious blend of simplicity and sophistication, making it a perfect choice for both everyday dining and special occasions.

Benefits:

1. Heart Health: Salmon is renowned for its high content of omega-3 fatty acids, which are known to promote cardiovascular health. Regular consumption may help lower the risk of heart

disease, reduce inflammation, and improve overall heart function.

2. Brain Boost: Omega-3s in salmon are also linked to cognitive health. They may enhance memory, concentration, and mood, making this dish a brain-boosting delight.

3. Protein Power: Salmon is an excellent source of high-quality protein, essential for muscle repair and overall body strength. It's a favorite among athletes and those looking to maintain a balanced diet.

Preparation:

Baking salmon with dill sauce is a straightforward yet elegant process. Season fresh salmon fillets with a pinch of salt, a dash of black pepper, and a squeeze of lemon juice. Then, place them in the oven and bake until the salmon flakes easily with a fork.

The dill sauce, a delightful companion to the salmon, is made by blending fresh dill, Greek yogurt, a touch of garlic, and lemon zest. Drizzle this creamy, herb-infused sauce over the baked salmon just before serving to elevate the dish to a new level of culinary delight.

In every succulent bite of baked salmon with dill sauce, you'll savor the marriage of exquisite flavors and the assurance of nourishing your body with a dish that supports your well-being. Whether it's a weeknight dinner or a special gathering, this recipe is a testament to the profound connection between good food and good health.

- GRILLED CHICKEN WITH LEMON-HERB MARINADE

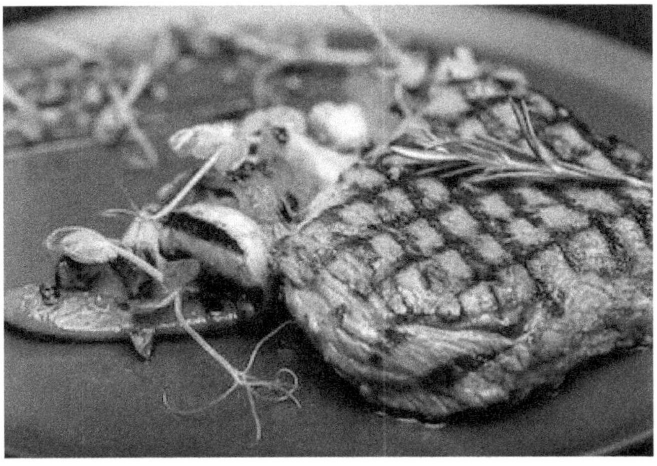

Grilled chicken with lemon-herb marinade is a culinary delight that marries health and flavor in a perfect union. This dish is not only a culinary masterpiece but also a testament to the benefits of wholesome cooking. Succulent, tender, and bursting with zesty goodness, it is a testament to how simple ingredients can transform an ordinary meal into a gastronomic experience.

Benefits:

- Lean Protein: Grilled chicken is an excellent source of lean protein, vital for muscle growth and repair, making it a nutritious choice for those seeking to maintain or improve their overall health.

- Low in Saturated Fat: This dish is naturally low in saturated fats, promoting heart health and reducing the risk of cardiovascular diseases.

- Rich in Flavor: The lemon-herb marinade not only enhances the taste but also provides a dose of antioxidants and vitamins, contributing to immune support and overall vitality.

- Versatility: Grilled chicken with lemon-herb marinade is versatile, making it a go-to option for weeknight dinners, family gatherings, or outdoor barbecues.

Preparation:

Marinating chicken in a blend of fresh lemon juice, aromatic herbs like rosemary, thyme, and oregano, along with minced garlic and olive oil, infuses the meat with a harmonious blend of citrusy, earthy flavors. After marinating for at least 30 minutes, the chicken is then grilled to perfection, achieving a tantalizing combination of smokiness and juiciness.

Grilled chicken with lemon-herb marinade is a testament to the culinary magic that happens when simplicity meets sophistication. It is not just a meal; it is an experience—a nourishing, delectable journey for the taste buds and a celebration of the many benefits of mindful eating.

- VEGETABLE STIR-FRY WITH TOFU

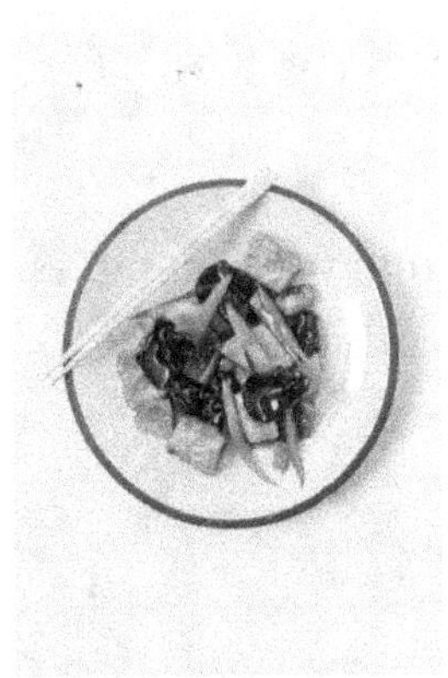

Vegetable stir-fry with tofu is a vibrant and wholesome dish that embodies the essence of healthy eating. Bursting with an array of colorful vegetables and plant-based protein, this stir-fry offers a delightful fusion of flavors and textures.

Benefits:

1. Nutrient-Rich: Tofu, a soy-based protein, is a nutritional powerhouse. It's low in saturated fat and an excellent source of essential amino acids, iron, and calcium. Coupled with an assortment of vegetables, this dish provides an abundance of vitamins, minerals, and antioxidants.

2. Heart-Healthy: The absence of saturated fats and cholesterol in tofu, combined with the heart-protective properties of vegetables, makes this stir-fry a heart-healthy choice. The inclusion of tofu in a plant-based diet has been associated with reduced cardiovascular risk.

3. Digestive Support: The fiber from the vegetables aids in digestion, while the probiotics found in fermented tofu varieties may contribute to a healthy gut microbiome.

Preparation:

Creating a vegetable stir-fry with tofu is both simple and versatile. Start by pressing and cubing extra-firm tofu to enhance its texture. Then, heat a wok or large skillet with a touch of oil and stir-fry your choice of vegetables, such as bell peppers, broccoli, carrots, and snap peas. Add tofu cubes and your preferred stir-fry sauce, like soy sauce or a savory sesame-ginger blend. Toss everything together until the tofu absorbs the flavors and the vegetables reach the desired tenderness. Serve your masterpiece over a bed of brown rice or noodles for a complete, satisfying meal that celebrates both taste and nutrition. Whether you're a seasoned cook or just beginning your culinary journey, vegetable stir-fry with tofu is a versatile, nutrient-packed delight that's sure to become a staple in your kitchen.

- LENTIL AND MUSHROOM STUFFED PEPPERS

Lentil and Mushroom Stuffed Peppers are a delightful fusion of flavors and textures that not only tantalize the taste buds but also provide a wealth of nutritional benefits. This vegetarian dish combines the earthy richness of mushrooms, the protein-packed goodness of lentils, and the vibrant sweetness of bell peppers, creating a symphony of tastes and colors on your plate.

Benefits:

- Nutrient-Rich: Lentils are a nutritional powerhouse, offering plant-based protein, fiber, vitamins, and minerals. They promote heart health, aid in digestion, and help regulate blood sugar levels.

- Mushroom Magic: Mushrooms provide an umami depth to the dish while delivering essential nutrients like vitamin D, selenium, and antioxidants. They support immune function and overall well-being.

- Low in Calories: Stuffed peppers are a satisfying, low-calorie option for those looking to maintain a healthy weight. The combination of lentils and vegetables helps you feel full without excessive calories.

- Dietary Flexibility: This dish is not only vegetarian but also vegan-friendly, making it suitable for a wide range of dietary preferences.

Preparation:

- Begin by selecting fresh bell peppers of your choice, preferably red, yellow, or green for their vibrant colors and sweet flavor.

- Prepare a filling by sautéing chopped mushrooms, onions, garlic, and cooked lentils with your favorite seasonings. You can also add herbs like thyme or rosemary for extra aroma.

- Carefully stuff the hollowed-out bell peppers with the lentil and mushroom mixture.

- Bake in the oven until the peppers are tender and slightly charred, creating a mouthwatering aroma.

- Garnish with fresh herbs or grated Parmesan cheese for an extra layer of flavor.

CHAPTER 6

SIDES AND SNACKS

These culinary companions can be both delicious and supportive of liver health, offering a world of exciting possibilities for those managing hepatitis. In this section, we explore an array of sides and snacks thoughtfully designed to nourish the body while ensuring the liver's well-being remains a top priority.

From wholesome sides that complement your main courses to satisfying snacks that satisfy cravings in a healthful manner, this chapter offers a range of options that embrace the principles of a hepatitis-friendly diet. By focusing on portion control, limiting sodium, and selecting ingredients that promote digestion and liver function, you can savor every bite with confidence. Whether you're enjoying roasted sweet potato wedges, a refreshing cucumber and Greek yogurt dip, or a handful of nutty brown rice cakes, these recipes and ideas are tailored to enhance your culinary journey while supporting your liver's vitality. So, let's embark on a flavorful exploration of sides and snacks that harmonize with hepatitis management, proving that a liver-conscious diet can be both nourishing and delicious.

- ROASTED SWEET POTATO WEDGES

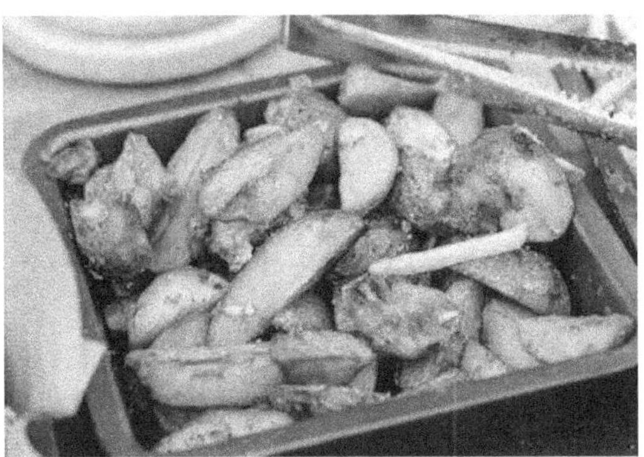

Roasted sweet potato wedges are not only a delectable addition to your meal but also a nutritional powerhouse that can elevate your culinary experience while supporting your well-being. These vibrant, orange-hued wedges are a delightful combination of wholesome taste and health benefits, making them a popular choice for health-conscious individuals and food enthusiasts alike.

Benefits:

- Rich in Vitamins and Minerals: Sweet potatoes are brimming with essential nutrients such as vitamin

A, vitamin C, and potassium, which bolster your immune system and promote heart health.

- Fiber and Digestive Health: Their fiber content aids digestion, keeps you feeling full, and supports a healthy gut, all while helping regulate blood sugar levels.

- Antioxidant Properties: Sweet potatoes are abundant in antioxidants, including beta-carotene, which combat oxidative stress and reduce the risk of chronic diseases.

- Satiety and Weight Management: These wedges offer a satisfyingly hearty texture, making them a satiating option that can assist in weight management.

Preparation:

Creating roasted sweet potato wedges is a simple and customizable process. Begin by washing, peeling (if desired), and cutting sweet potatoes into wedges or strips. Toss them with a touch of olive oil, salt, and your preferred seasonings, such as paprika, rosemary, or cinnamon, for added flavor. Then, roast them in the oven until they achieve a crispy exterior and tender interior. The versatility of sweet potato wedges allows you to experiment with various herbs and spices to suit your palate, making them a versatile and healthful addition to any meal.

Whether served as a side dish or a satisfying snack, roasted sweet potato wedges are a delightful culinary choice that offers both flavor and nourishment, adding vibrancy and nutritional value to your plate.

- HUMMUS WITH FRESH VEGETABLES

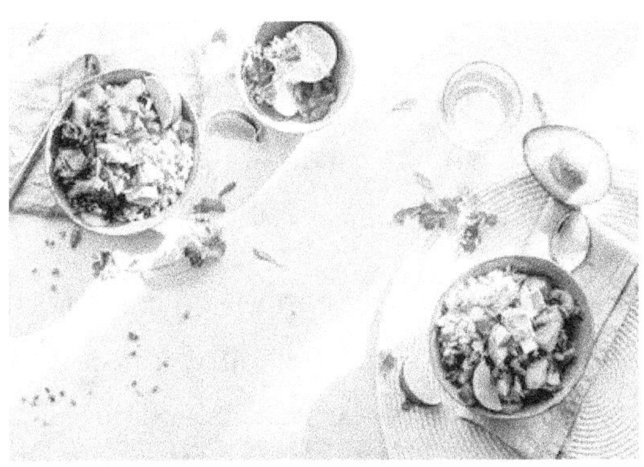

Hummus, the velvety Middle Eastern dip made from creamy chickpeas, tahini, and a burst of aromatic flavors, is a culinary treasure that has gained international popularity for good reason. Paired with fresh vegetables, it transforms into a wholesome and delectable snack or appetizer, offering a symphony of flavors and a plethora of health benefits.

Benefits:

- Nutrient-Rich: Hummus is a nutritional powerhouse, packed with plant-based protein, fiber, and essential vitamins and minerals. Chickpeas provide a protein source that supports muscle health and helps keep you feeling full and satisfied.

- Heart-Healthy: The ingredients in hummus, such as olive oil and tahini, contribute healthy fats, including monounsaturated fats and omega-3 fatty acids. These fats have been linked to improved heart health and reduced inflammation.

- Digestive Wellness: The fiber content in chickpeas aids in digestion and promotes a healthy gut. It can alleviate constipation and support a balanced digestive system.

Preparation:

Making hummus with fresh vegetables is a breeze. Start with a classic hummus base by blending chickpeas, tahini, lemon juice, garlic, and olive oil until smooth. Season with salt, pepper, and a pinch of cumin for depth of flavor.

For the fresh vegetables, choose an assortment of colorful options like cucumber slices, cherry tomatoes, carrot sticks, bell pepper strips, and celery. These vegetables not only add vibrant colors but also offer a variety of vitamins, minerals, and antioxidants to further boost the nutritional value of your snack.

Hummus with fresh vegetables is a culinary delight that balances indulgence with nutrition. Whether as a wholesome snack, a party appetizer, or a light meal, it's a versatile and delicious option that caters to your taste buds and nourishes your body.

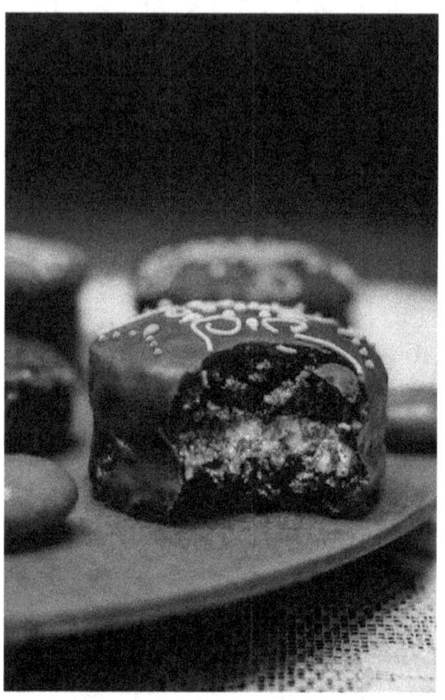

Brown rice cakes with nut butter are a simple yet nourishing snack that has gained popularity for its delightful taste and remarkable health benefits. Combining the wholesome goodness of brown rice cakes with the richness of nut butter, this snack offers a satisfying and nutritious option for those seeking a quick energy boost, a source of healthy fats, and a dose of essential nutrients.

Benefits:

1. Nutrient-Packed: Brown rice cakes provide complex carbohydrates and dietary fiber, offering sustained energy and aiding digestion. Nut butter, whether almond, peanut, or cashew, delivers heart-healthy monounsaturated fats, plant-based protein, and essential vitamins and minerals like vitamin E and magnesium.

2. Satiety and Weight Management: The combination of fiber and healthy fats in brown rice cakes with nut butter can promote feelings of fullness, making it an excellent choice for curbing cravings and supporting weight management.

3. Heart Health: Monounsaturated fats found in nut butter are known to improve cardiovascular health by reducing bad cholesterol levels. Additionally, the magnesium content helps regulate blood pressure.

Preparation:

Creating this wholesome snack is quick and effortless:

- Start with high-quality brown rice cakes and your choice of nut butter.

- Spread a generous layer of nut butter evenly onto each rice cake.

- Customize with additional toppings such as sliced bananas, honey, or a sprinkle of chia seeds for added texture and flavor.

Brown rice cakes with nut butter are a versatile and convenient snack suitable for any time of day. Whether enjoyed as a pre-workout boost or a mid-afternoon pick-me-up, they offer a delicious way to nourish your body and satisfy your taste buds while reaping the health benefits of whole grains and nutrient-rich nut butter.

- CUCUMBER AND GREEK YOGURT DIP

Cucumber and Greek Yogurt Dip, often affectionately known as "Tzatziki," is a delectable and healthful addition to any culinary repertoire. This refreshing dip is not only a flavorful accompaniment but also a nutritional powerhouse, offering a multitude of benefits to those seeking a delightful and wholesome snack or condiment.

Benefits:

- Rich in Protein: Greek yogurt, the star ingredient, boasts a high protein content, which can help promote muscle health and satiety.

- Low in Calories: This dip is waistline-friendly, making it an ideal choice for those mindful of calorie intake.

- Probiotic Boost: Greek yogurt is rich in probiotics, beneficial bacteria that support gut health and digestion.

- Hydrating and Nutrient-Rich: Cucumbers are predominantly composed of water and offer vitamins and minerals, including potassium and vitamins K and C.

- Cooling and Refreshing: The combination of yogurt and cucumber creates a cooling effect, making it an ideal choice for hot days or as a complement to spicy dishes.

Preparation:

Making Cucumber and Greek Yogurt Dip is a breeze. Start by finely grating cucumbers and draining excess moisture. Mix them with Greek yogurt, minced garlic, fresh dill or mint, a dash of olive oil, and a squeeze of lemon juice. Season with salt and pepper to taste. Refrigerate for at least an hour to allow the flavors to meld, and voila! Serve it with pita bread, as a dip for veggies, or as a condiment for grilled meats.

This versatile dip not only tantalizes the taste buds but also nourishes the body, making it a must-have recipe in any kitchen. Cucumber and Greek Yogurt Dip is the cool and creamy solution.

CHAPTER 7

SWEETS AND TREATS

Indulging in delectable sweets and treats need not be off-limits when managing hepatitis. In fact, crafting nourishing and liver-friendly desserts can be a delightful part of a well-rounded dietary approach. This chapter, "Sweets and Treats," invites you to explore a world of delicious, yet health-conscious, options designed to satisfy your sweet cravings while supporting your liver.

- BANANA AND ALMOND BUTTER COOKIES

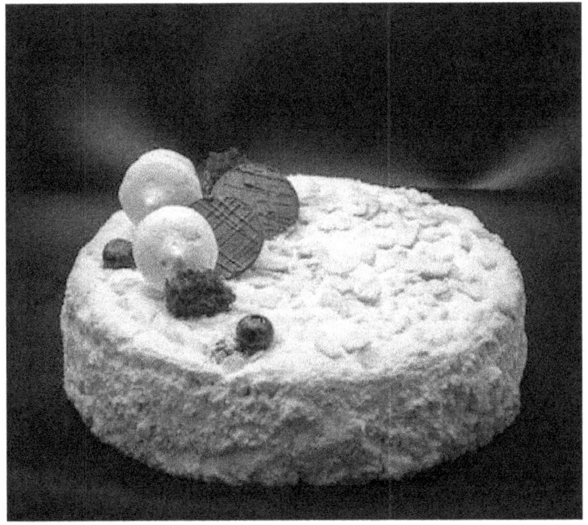

Banana and almond butter cookies offer a delightful twist on the classic treat, combining the natural sweetness of ripe bananas with the creamy richness of almond butter. These cookies are not only a delicious indulgence but also a healthier alternative, as they are typically low in added sugars and packed with nutritional benefits. They make for a perfect guilt-free snack or a wholesome dessert option.

Preparation:

1. Ingredients:

   - 2 ripe bananas, mashed

   - 1/2 cup almond butter

   - 1 teaspoon vanilla extract

   - 1 cup rolled oats

   - 1/4 cup almond flour

   - 1/2 teaspoon baking powder

   - 1/2 teaspoon cinnamon (optional)

   - A pinch of salt

2. Mix Wet Ingredients: In a mixing bowl, combine the mashed bananas, almond butter, and vanilla extract. Mix until you have a smooth, creamy mixture.

3. Add Dry Ingredients: Stir in the rolled oats, almond flour, baking powder, cinnamon (if desired), and a pinch of salt. Mix until all the ingredients are well combined.

4. Form Cookies: Drop spoonfuls of the cookie dough onto a baking sheet lined with parchment paper. Use the back of a fork to flatten and shape each cookie.

5. Bake: Preheat your oven to 350°F (175°C). Bake the cookies for about 10-12 minutes or until they are golden brown.

6. Cool and Enjoy: Allow the cookies to cool on a wire rack for a few minutes before indulging in their chewy, nutty, and naturally sweet goodness.

These banana and almond butter cookies are a testament to how healthy ingredients can come together to create a scrumptious treat. Enjoy them guilt-free as a satisfying snack or dessert that's both nutritious and delicious.

- BERRY PARFAIT WITH YOGURT

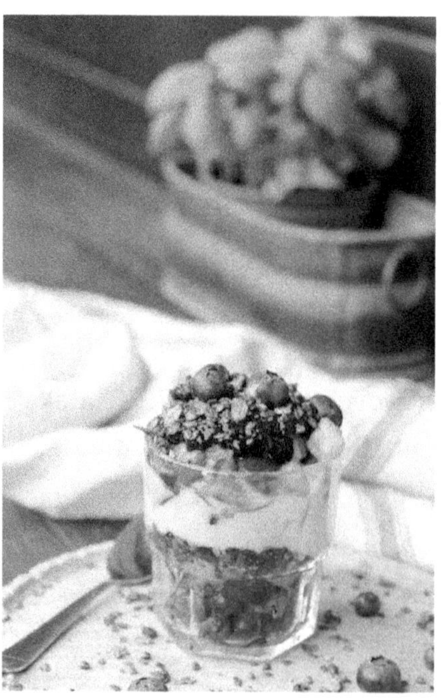

A tantalizing treat that not only satisfies your taste buds but also offers a plethora of health benefits. This wholesome concoction combines the creamy goodness of yogurt with the vibrant, natural sweetness of berries, creating a symphony of flavors and textures that are as nourishing as they are delicious.

Benefits:

- Rich in Antioxidants: Berries, such as blueberries, strawberries, and raspberries, are packed with antioxidants that combat free radicals, promoting overall health and potentially reducing the risk of chronic diseases.

- Protein and Probiotics: Yogurt serves as an excellent source of protein and probiotics, supporting digestive health, aiding in weight management, and contributing to a strong immune system.

- Bone Health: Yogurt is rich in calcium and vitamin D, essential for maintaining strong bones and preventing osteoporosis.

Preparation:

Creating a Berry Parfait with Yogurt is a breeze. Begin by layering a serving of creamy yogurt with a handful of fresh, washed berries in a glass or bowl. Repeat the layers to your liking, and consider adding a drizzle of honey for a touch of natural sweetness. Garnish with some chopped nuts or a sprinkle of granola for added crunch and nutrition.

This delectable Berry Parfait with Yogurt not only satiates your dessert cravings but also nourishes your body with a medley of vitamins, minerals, and antioxidants, making it an ideal choice for a health-conscious and flavor-loving palate. Enjoy it as a breakfast option, snack, or even as a guilt-free dessert to treat yourself to a burst of vitality.

- DARK CHOCOLATE-DIPPED STRAWBERRIES

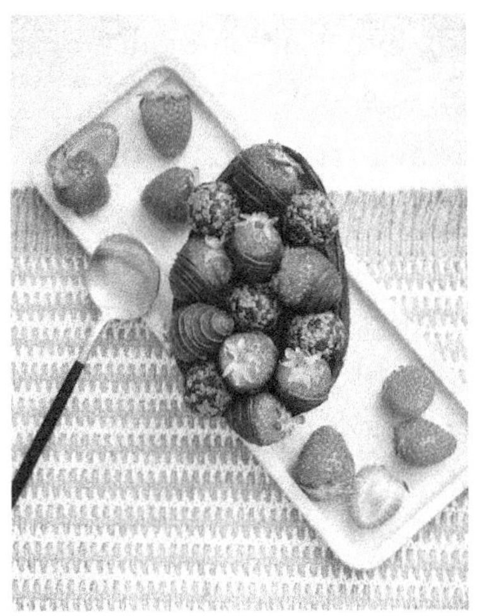

Indulgent and healthful, dark chocolate-dipped strawberries combine two delightful worlds of flavor in one exquisite bite. These delectable treats offer a delightful balance between the richness of dark chocolate and the natural sweetness of ripe strawberries. As a dessert that marries taste with potential health benefits, dark chocolate-dipped strawberries have become a favorite for those seeking both a guilt-free indulgence and a dose of antioxidants.

Benefits:

Dark chocolate is known for its antioxidant properties, which can help combat free radicals and support heart health. It may also enhance mood and brain function due to its serotonin-boosting compounds. Strawberries, on the other hand, are a vitamin C powerhouse and are low in calories, making them a nutritious choice for a sweet treat. When combined, these two ingredients create a dessert that's not only satisfying to the palate but also offers potential health perks.

Preparation:

To create dark chocolate-dipped strawberries, begin by melting high-quality dark chocolate in a microwave or over a double boiler. Then, dip each washed and dried strawberry into the melted chocolate, ensuring even coverage. Place the dipped strawberries on parchment paper and let them cool until the chocolate hardens. For an extra touch of sophistication, drizzle some additional melted dark chocolate over the top. Enjoy these delectable creations as a dessert, snack, or even as an elegant addition to special occasions. Whether it's a romantic gesture or a self-indulgent moment, dark chocolate-dipped strawberries are a delightful choice that combines flavor, health benefits, and sheer culinary pleasure.

- CHIA SEED PUDDING WITH MIXED NUTS

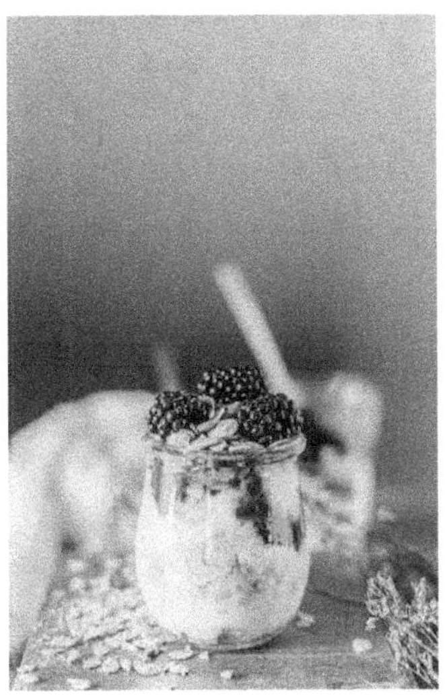

Chia seed pudding with mixed nuts is a delectable and wholesome treat that not only tantalizes the taste buds but also offers a myriad of health benefits. This creamy and satisfying pudding combines the nutritional prowess of chia seeds, the crunch of mixed nuts, and a touch of sweetness for a delightful and nutritious dessert or breakfast option.

Benefits:

- Omega-3 Fatty Acids: Chia seeds are a rich source of heart-healthy omega-3 fatty acids, which can help reduce inflammation and support cardiovascular health.

- Fiber-Rich: Chia seeds are packed with soluble fiber, promoting digestive regularity and providing a feeling of fullness that aids in weight management.

- Protein Power: Mixed nuts add an extra protein punch, helping to build and repair tissues while keeping hunger at bay.

- Antioxidant Boost: Nuts provide essential antioxidants, protecting cells from oxidative damage and supporting overall well-being.

Preparation:

Creating chia seed pudding with mixed nuts is a breeze. Simply mix chia seeds with your choice of milk (dairy or plant-based) and sweetener (such as honey or maple syrup), then refrigerate for a few hours or overnight until it reaches a pudding-like consistency. Top with a medley of mixed nuts, including almonds, walnuts, and cashews, for added texture and flavor. This versatile dish can be customized with your favorite toppings like fresh berries, sliced bananas, or a sprinkle of cinnamon.

Whether enjoyed as a healthy dessert or a nutrient-packed breakfast, chia seed pudding with mixed nuts is a delightful way to nourish your body and indulge your taste buds.

CHAPTER 8

BEVERAGES FOR LIVER HEALTH

The health of our liver is vital to our overall well-being, as this remarkable organ performs numerous critical functions, from detoxifying the body to aiding in digestion. Choosing the right beverages can significantly impact liver health, helping it function optimally and potentially preventing liver-related issues. In this exploration of "Beverages for Liver Health," we delve into the world of liquid nourishment, unveiling a spectrum of drinks that can benefit the liver and the body as a whole.

From refreshing detox waters infused with natural ingredients to herbal teas renowned for their cleansing properties, this journey through beverages will empower you to make informed choices that support and protect your liver. Whether you're seeking to enhance liver function, prevent liver disease, or simply promote overall wellness, this guide will introduce you to a variety of beverages that can be incorporated into your daily routine. Join us as we sip our way to better liver health, one refreshing and healthful beverage at a time.

- LEMON WATER DETOX DRINK

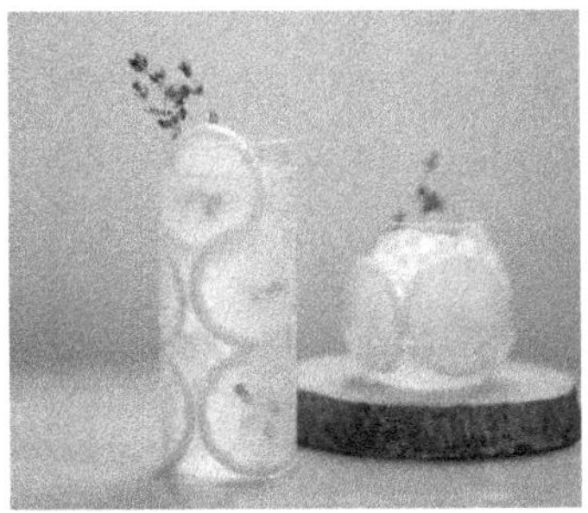

Lemon water detox drink, often touted as a morning elixir, is a simple yet powerful concoction that has gained popularity for its numerous health benefits and refreshing taste. This revitalizing beverage is made by combining freshly squeezed lemon juice with water, creating a natural and low-calorie detoxification aid that can kickstart your day on a healthy note.

Benefits:

Lemon water detox offers an array of health advantages:

- Detoxification: Lemon's high vitamin C content supports liver function, aiding in the removal of toxins and promoting overall detoxification.

- Hydration: Staying adequately hydrated is vital for digestion, metabolism, and maintaining healthy skin, and lemon water provides a flavorful way to increase daily water intake.

- Digestive Health: Lemon water stimulates the production of digestive enzymes, potentially improving digestion and alleviating symptoms like bloating and indigestion.

- Weight Management: Some studies suggest that lemon water may help control appetite and support weight loss efforts when part of a balanced diet.

- Boosted Immunity: Vitamin C and antioxidants in lemons bolster the immune system, potentially reducing the risk of illnesses.

Preparation:

To prepare lemon water detox drink, simply:

- Squeeze the juice of half a lemon into a glass of warm or room temperature water.

- Optionally, add a drizzle of honey or a pinch of cayenne pepper for flavor variations.

- Stir well and enjoy it in the morning on an empty stomach for maximum benefits.

Incorporating lemon water detox into your daily routine can be a refreshing way to promote overall well-being and kickstart your day with a burst of vitality. However, it's essential to remember that while lemon water offers many advantages, it should be part of a balanced diet and a healthy lifestyle.

- GREEN TEA WITH HONEY AND LEMON

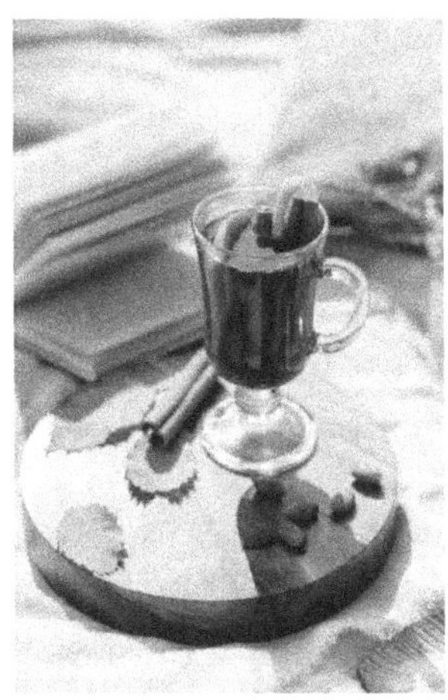

Green tea with honey and lemon is more than just a soothing beverage; it's a delightful elixir that offers a wealth of health benefits. This concoction combines the earthy notes of green tea with the sweetness of honey and the zesty tang of lemon, creating a harmonious blend that not only tantalizes the taste buds but also promotes overall wellness.

Benefits:

- Antioxidant Powerhouse: Green tea is renowned for its high levels of antioxidants, particularly catechins, which help combat oxidative stress and reduce the risk of chronic diseases.

- Digestive Aid: The addition of lemon in this brew may support digestion and alleviate indigestion, making it a gentle yet effective digestive aid.

- Immune Support: Honey is known for its antibacterial and anti-inflammatory properties, potentially boosting the immune system and providing relief from sore throats.

- Metabolic Boost: Green tea has been linked to increased metabolism and fat oxidation, making it a helpful addition to weight management efforts.

Preparation:

- Boil water and allow it to cool slightly, ideally to about 180°F (82°C), as boiling water can make green tea bitter.

- Add a green tea bag or loose tea leaves to a cup.

- Pour the hot (but not boiling) water over the tea and steep for 2-3 minutes.

- Remove the tea bag or strain the leaves.

- Squeeze in fresh lemon juice and add honey to taste.

- Stir well and enjoy this invigorating beverage, either hot or chilled.

This green tea infusion is not only a delightful daily ritual but also a flavorful way to support your overall well-being. Whether you savor it in the morning to kickstart your day or as an afternoon pick-me-up, green tea with honey and lemon offers a refreshing and healthful escape from the ordinary.

- LIVER-BOOSTING SMOOTHIES

Liver-boosting smoothies are a delicious and healthful way to fortify your body's natural detoxification powerhouse – the liver. These vibrant concoctions are designed to not only tantalize your taste buds but also provide a plethora of benefits for your liver's well-being.

Benefits:

- Liver Cleansing: The ingredients in liver-boosting smoothies often include antioxidants, vitamins, and minerals that help flush out toxins from the liver, promoting a cleaner and more efficient detoxification process.

- Nutrient-Packed: These smoothies are bursting with nutrients like vitamin C, which supports liver function, and fiber, which aids digestion and prevents the buildup of harmful substances.

- Inflammation Reduction: Many ingredients possess anti-inflammatory properties, such as turmeric and ginger, which can help soothe liver inflammation and enhance its resilience.

Preparation:

Creating liver-boosting smoothies is a breeze. Simply blend together a variety of liver-loving ingredients such as leafy greens (like spinach or kale), citrus fruits (like lemon or orange), antioxidant-rich berries, detoxifying herbs (like parsley or cilantro), and healthy fats (such as avocado or flaxseed oil).

- HERBAL INFUSIONS AND TINCTURES

Herbal infusions and tinctures are age-old remedies that harness the power of nature's botanical treasures to promote health and well-being. These liquid concoctions offer a holistic approach to healing, blending the therapeutic benefits of herbs, roots, and flowers with the art of preparation.

Benefits:

These herbal elixirs hold a myriad of potential benefits. Infusions, typically prepared by steeping herbs in hot water, provide a gentle and soothing way to extract essential compounds that can aid digestion, ease stress, and boost immunity. Tinctures, on the other hand, concentrate the healing properties of herbs in alcohol or glycerin, offering a potent solution that may alleviate ailments such as insomnia, anxiety, or digestive discomfort.

Preparation:

To craft herbal infusions, dried or fresh herbs are steeped in hot water for a specified period. Popular choices include chamomile for relaxation or peppermint for digestive relief. Tinctures require a longer preparation process, involving maceration and aging to intensify the herb's potency.

CHAPTER 9

MEAL PLANS

Week 1: Hepatitis-Friendly Meal Plan

Day 1:

- Breakfast: Oatmeal topped with sliced bananas and a drizzle of honey.

- Snack: Greek yogurt with a handful of mixed berries.

- Lunch: Grilled chicken breast with quinoa and steamed broccoli.

- Snack: Sliced cucumber with hummus.

- Dinner: Baked salmon with brown rice and roasted asparagus.

Day 2:

- Breakfast: Scrambled eggs with spinach and cherry tomatoes.

- Snack: A small apple with a tablespoon of almond butter.

- Lunch: Lentil soup with a side salad of mixed greens.

- Snack: Mixed nuts.

- Dinner: Grilled shrimp with quinoa and sautéed zucchini.

Day 3:

- Breakfast: Smoothie with spinach, banana, and low-fat Greek yogurt.

- Snack: Sliced carrots with tzatziki sauce.

- Lunch: Turkey and avocado whole-grain wrap with a side of mixed greens.

- Snack: Cottage cheese with pineapple chunks.

- Dinner: Baked cod with brown rice and steamed green beans.

Day 4:

- Breakfast: Greek yogurt parfait with low-sugar granola and fresh strawberries.

- Snack: Sliced bell peppers with hummus.

- Lunch: Spinach and feta stuffed chicken breast with a side of quinoa.

- Snack: Celery sticks with peanut butter.

- Dinner: Beef stir-fry with broccoli and brown rice.

Day 5:

- Breakfast: Omelet with low-fat cheese, tomatoes, and bell peppers.

- Snack: Sliced pear with a sprinkle of cinnamon.

- Lunch: Grilled vegetable salad with chickpeas and balsamic vinaigrette.

- Snack: A handful of cherry tomatoes with balsamic vinegar.

- Dinner: Baked tilapia with quinoa and roasted Brussels sprouts.

Day 6:

- Breakfast: Whole-grain pancakes with a small portion of blueberries.

- Snack: Mixed nuts.

- Lunch: Tofu and vegetable stir-fry with brown rice.

- Snack: Baby carrots with tzatziki sauce.

- Dinner: Chicken and vegetable kebabs with couscous.

Day 7:

- Breakfast: Scrambled egg whites with sautéed spinach and whole-grain toast.

- Snack: Low-fat cottage cheese with pineapple.

- Lunch: Spinach and mushroom quiche with a side salad.

- Snack: Sliced cucumber with hummus.

- Dinner: Pork tenderloin with mashed cauliflower and steamed broccoli.

Week 2: Hepatitis-Friendly Meal Plan

Day 1:

- Breakfast: Oatmeal with sliced bananas and a drizzle of honey.

- Snack: Greek yogurt with a handful of mixed berries.

- Lunch: Grilled chicken breast with quinoa and steamed broccoli.

- Snack: Sliced cucumber with hummus.

- Dinner: Baked salmon with brown rice and roasted asparagus.

Day 2:

- Breakfast: Scrambled eggs with spinach and cherry tomatoes.

- Snack: A small apple with a tablespoon of almond butter.

- Lunch: Lentil soup with a side salad of mixed greens.

- Snack: Mixed nuts.

- Dinner: Grilled shrimp with quinoa and sautéed zucchini.

Day 3:

- Breakfast: Smoothie with spinach, banana, and low-fat Greek yogurt.

- Snack: Sliced carrots with tzatziki sauce.

- Lunch: Turkey and avocado whole-grain wrap with a side of mixed greens.

- Snack: Cottage cheese with pineapple chunks.

- Dinner: Baked cod with brown rice and steamed green beans.

Day 4:

- Breakfast: Greek yogurt parfait with low-sugar granola and fresh strawberries.

- Snack: Sliced bell peppers with hummus.

- Lunch: Spinach and feta stuffed chicken breast with a side of quinoa.

- Snack: Celery sticks with peanut butter.

- Dinner: Beef stir-fry with broccoli and brown rice.

Day 5:

- Breakfast: Omelet with low-fat cheese, tomatoes, and bell peppers.

- Snack: Sliced pear with a sprinkle of cinnamon.

- Lunch: Grilled vegetable salad with chickpeas and balsamic vinaigrette.

- Snack: A handful of cherry tomatoes with balsamic vinegar.

- Dinner: Baked tilapia with quinoa and roasted Brussels sprouts.

Day 6:

- Breakfast: Whole-grain pancakes with a small portion of blueberries.

- Snack: Mixed nuts.

- Lunch: Tofu and vegetable stir-fry with brown rice.

- Snack: Baby carrots with tzatziki sauce.

- Dinner: Chicken and vegetable kebabs with couscous.

Day 7:

- Breakfast: Scrambled egg whites with sautéed spinach and whole-grain toast.

- Snack: Low-fat cottage cheese with pineapple.

- Lunch: Spinach and mushroom quiche with a side salad.

- Snack: Sliced cucumber with hummus.

- Dinner: Pork tenderloin with mashed cauliflower and steamed broccoli.

Week 3: Hepatitis-Friendly Meal Plan

Day 1:

- Breakfast: Oatmeal topped with sliced bananas and a drizzle of honey.

- Snack: Greek yogurt with a handful of mixed berries.

- Lunch: Grilled chicken breast with quinoa and steamed broccoli.

- Snack: Sliced cucumber with hummus.

- Dinner: Baked salmon with brown rice and roasted asparagus.

Day 2:

- Breakfast: Scrambled eggs with spinach and cherry tomatoes.

- Snack: A small apple with a tablespoon of almond butter.

- Lunch: Lentil soup with a side salad of mixed greens.

- Snack: Mixed nuts.

- Dinner: Grilled shrimp with quinoa and sautéed zucchini.

Day 3:

- Breakfast: Smoothie with spinach, banana, and low-fat Greek yogurt.

- Snack: Sliced carrots with tzatziki sauce.

- Lunch: Turkey and avocado whole-grain wrap with a side of mixed greens.

- Snack: Cottage cheese with pineapple chunks.

- Dinner: Baked cod with brown rice and steamed green beans.

Day 4:

- Breakfast: Greek yogurt parfait with low-sugar granola and fresh strawberries.

- Snack: Sliced bell peppers with hummus.

- Lunch: Spinach and feta stuffed chicken breast with a side of quinoa.

- Snack: Celery sticks with peanut butter.

- Dinner: Beef stir-fry with broccoli and brown rice.

Day 5:

- Breakfast: Omelet with low-fat cheese, tomatoes, and bell peppers.

- Snack: Sliced pear with a sprinkle of cinnamon.

- Lunch: Grilled vegetable salad with chickpeas and balsamic vinaigrette.

- Snack: A handful of cherry tomatoes with balsamic vinegar.

- Dinner: Baked tilapia with quinoa and roasted Brussels sprouts.

Day 6:

- Breakfast: Whole-grain pancakes with a small portion of blueberries.

- Snack: Mixed nuts.

- Lunch: Tofu and vegetable stir-fry with brown rice.

- Snack: Baby carrots with tzatziki sauce.

- Dinner: Chicken and vegetable kebabs with couscous.

Day 7:

- Breakfast: Scrambled egg whites with sautéed spinach and whole-grain toast.

- Snack: Low-fat cottage cheese with pineapple.

- Lunch: Spinach and mushroom quiche with a side salad.

- Snack: Sliced cucumber with hummus.

- Dinner: Pork tenderloin with mashed cauliflower and steamed broccoli.

Week 4: Hepatitis-Friendly Meal Plan

Day 1:

- Breakfast: Oatmeal topped with sliced bananas and a drizzle of honey.

- Snack: Greek yogurt with a handful of mixed berries.

- Lunch: Grilled chicken breast with quinoa and steamed broccoli.

- Snack: Sliced cucumber with hummus.

- Dinner: Baked salmon with brown rice and roasted asparagus.

Day 2:

- Breakfast: Scrambled eggs with spinach and cherry tomatoes.

- Snack: A small apple with a tablespoon of almond butter.

- Lunch: Lentil soup with a side salad of mixed greens.

- Snack: Mixed nuts.

- Dinner: Grilled shrimp with quinoa and sautéed zucchini.

Day 3:

- Breakfast: Smoothie with spinach, banana, and low-fat Greek yogurt.

- Snack: Sliced carrots with tzatziki sauce.

- Lunch: Turkey and avocado whole-grain wrap with a side of mixed greens.

- Snack: Cottage cheese with pineapple chunks.

- Dinner: Baked cod with brown rice and steamed green beans.

Day 4:

- Breakfast: Greek yogurt parfait with low-sugar granola and fresh strawberries.

- Snack: Sliced bell peppers with hummus.

- Lunch: Spinach and feta stuffed chicken breast with a side of quinoa.

- Snack: Celery sticks with peanut butter.

- Dinner: Beef stir-fry with broccoli and brown rice.

Day 5:

- Breakfast: Omelet with low-fat cheese, tomatoes, and bell peppers.

- Snack: Sliced pear with a sprinkle of cinnamon.

- Lunch: Grilled vegetable salad with chickpeas and balsamic vinaigrette.

- Snack: A handful of cherry tomatoes with balsamic vinegar.

- Dinner: Baked tilapia with quinoa and roasted Brussels sprouts.

Day 6:

- Breakfast: Whole-grain pancakes with a small portion of blueberries.

- Snack: Mixed nuts.

- Lunch: Tofu and vegetable stir-fry with brown rice.

- Snack: Baby carrots with tzatziki sauce.

- Dinner: Chicken and vegetable kebabs with couscous.

Day 7:

- Breakfast: Scrambled egg whites with sautéed spinach and whole-grain toast.

- Snack: Low-fat cottage cheese with pineapple.

- Lunch: Spinach and mushroom quiche with a side salad.

- Snack: Sliced cucumber with hummus.

- Dinner: Pork tenderloin with mashed cauliflower and steamed broccoli.

Week 4: Hepatitis-Friendly Meal Plan

Day 1:

- Breakfast: Oatmeal topped with sliced bananas and a drizzle of honey.

- Snack: Greek yogurt with a handful of mixed berries.

- Lunch: Grilled chicken breast with quinoa and steamed broccoli.

- Snack: Sliced cucumber with hummus.

- Dinner: Baked salmon with brown rice and roasted asparagus.

Day 2:

- Breakfast: Scrambled eggs with spinach and cherry tomatoes.

- Snack: A small apple with a tablespoon of almond butter.

- Lunch: Lentil soup with a side salad of mixed greens.

- Snack: Mixed nuts.

- Dinner: Grilled shrimp with quinoa and sautéed zucchini.

Day 3:

- Breakfast: Smoothie with spinach, banana, and low-fat Greek yogurt.

- Snack: Sliced carrots with tzatziki sauce.

- Lunch: Turkey and avocado whole-grain wrap with a side of mixed greens.

- Snack: Cottage cheese with pineapple chunks.

- Dinner: Baked cod with brown rice and steamed green beans.

Day 4:

- Breakfast: Greek yogurt parfait with low-sugar granola and fresh strawberries.

- Snack: Sliced bell peppers with hummus.

- Lunch: Spinach and feta stuffed chicken breast with a side of quinoa.

- Snack: Celery sticks with peanut butter.

- Dinner: Beef stir-fry with broccoli and brown rice.

Day 5:

- Breakfast: Omelet with low-fat cheese, tomatoes, and bell peppers.

- Snack: Sliced pear with a sprinkle of cinnamon.

- Lunch: Grilled vegetable salad with chickpeas and balsamic vinaigrette.

- Snack: A handful of cherry tomatoes with balsamic vinegar.

- Dinner: Baked tilapia with quinoa and roasted Brussels sprouts.

Day 6:

- Breakfast: Whole-grain pancakes with a small portion of blueberries.

- Snack: Mixed nuts.

- Lunch: Tofu and vegetable stir-fry with brown rice.

- Snack: Baby carrots with tzatziki sauce.

- Dinner: Chicken and vegetable kebabs with couscous.

Day 7:

- Breakfast: Scrambled egg whites with sautéed spinach and whole-grain toast.

- Snack: Low-fat cottage cheese with pineapple.

- Lunch: Spinach and mushroom quiche with a side salad.

- Snack: Sliced cucumber with hummus.

- Dinner: Pork tenderloin with mashed cauliflower and steamed broccoli.

CONCLUSION

Managing hepatitis through diet is a crucial aspect of maintaining liver health and overall well-being. Throughout this dietary journey, we've explored the importance of selecting foods that are gentle on the liver, reducing strain on this vital organ, and promoting a supportive environment for healing. From nutrient-dense meals to portion control, we've focused on crafting a diet tailored to the unique needs of individuals living with hepatitis.

However, it's essential to remember that diet is just one piece of the puzzle in the journey to living well with hepatitis. Beyond dietary choices, a holistic approach to health is paramount. This includes:

- Regular Medical Care: Continuously consult with healthcare providers who specialize in liver health. They can monitor your condition, adjust treatment plans, and provide essential guidance on managing hepatitis.

- Physical Activity: Incorporate regular, moderate exercise into your routine, as it can improve circulation, boost energy levels, and support overall health.

- Stress Management: Explore stress-reduction techniques such as mindfulness, meditation, or yoga, as chronic stress can exacerbate liver conditions.

- Medication Adherence: If prescribed medications, it's vital to take them as directed by your healthcare provider. Medications can play a crucial role in managing hepatitis.

- Avoiding Harmful Substances: Steer clear of alcohol, tobacco, and illicit drugs, as they can exacerbate liver damage.

- Supportive Network: Surround yourself with a strong support network, including friends and family who can provide emotional and practical support on your journey.

Additional Resources and References

In your quest for managing hepatitis and living a fulfilling life, there are numerous resources available to you. These resources offer further information, support, and a sense of community. Some valuable resources include:

- Hepatitis C Associations: National and international organizations dedicated to hepatitis, such as the American Liver Foundation, offer educational materials, support groups, and helplines.

- Liver Specialists: Consult with hepatologists or gastroenterologists who specialize in liver diseases for personalized care and guidance.

- Online Communities: Join online forums and communities where individuals living with hepatitis share their experiences, offer advice, and provide emotional support.

- Educational Materials: Libraries, websites, and healthcare institutions provide extensive educational materials on hepatitis management, treatment options, and the latest research.

- Clinical Trials: Explore opportunities to participate in clinical trials aimed at advancing hepatitis treatments and finding potential cures.

KEEP YOUR HEALTH SAFE

LEAVE A POSITIVE REVIEW ON THE AMAZON WEBSITE